# Diabetic Desserts, Juices & Smoothies

## An Unmissable Collection of Delicious Diabetic Sweets & Drinks to Enjoy Your Diabetic Diet

Valerie Blanchard

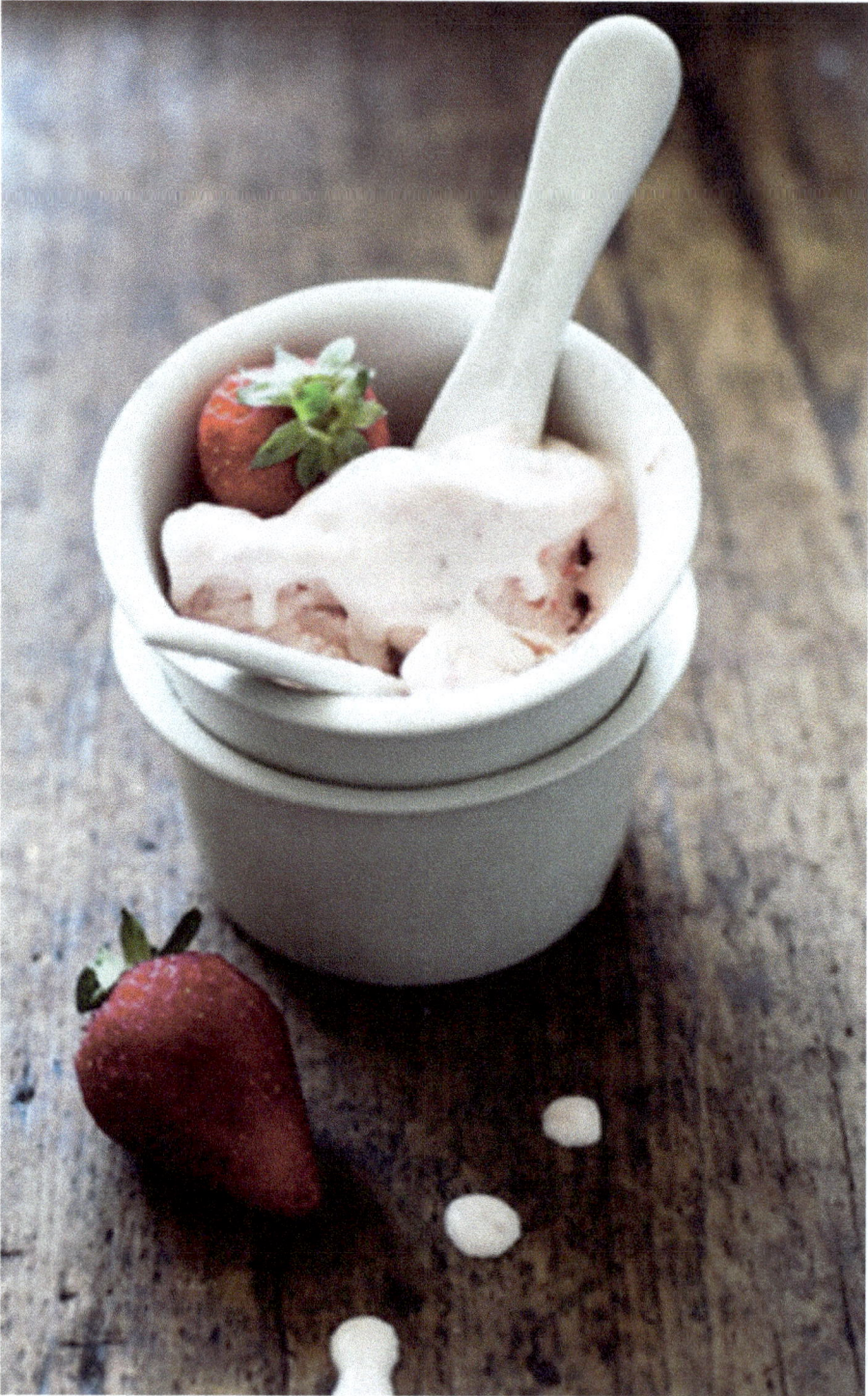

# Table of Contents

# Alkaline Raw Pumpkin Pie

***Preparation Time:*** 5 minutes

***Cooking Time***: 5 minutes

Servings: *4*

## Ingredients:

**Ingredients** for Pie Crust

- Cinnamon, one (1) teaspoon

- Dates/Turkish apricots, one (1) cup

- Raw almonds, one (1) cup

- Coconut flakes (unsweetened), one (1) cup

**Ingredients** for Pie Filling

- Dates, six (6)

- Cinnamon, ½ teaspoon

- Nutmeg, ½ teaspoon

- Pecans (soaked overnight), one (1) cup

- Organic pumpkin Blends (12 oz.), 1 ¼ cup

- Nutmeg, ½ teaspoon

- Sea salt (Himalayan or Celtic Sea Salt), ¼ teaspoon

- Vanilla, 1 teaspoon

- Gluten-free tamari

## *Directions:*

**Directions** for pie crust

1. Get a food processor and blend all the pie crust **Ingredients** at the same time.

2. Make sure the mixture turns oily and sticky before you stop mixing.

3. Put the mixture in a pie pan and mold against the sides and floor, to make it stick properly.

**Directions** for the pie filling

1. Mix **Ingredients** together in a blender.

2. Add the mixture to fill in the pie crust.

3. Pour some cinnamon on top.

4. Then refrigerate till it's cold.

5.  Then mold.


**_Nutrition:_** Calories 135; Calories from Fat 41.4; Total Fat 4.6 g; Cholesterol 11.3 mg

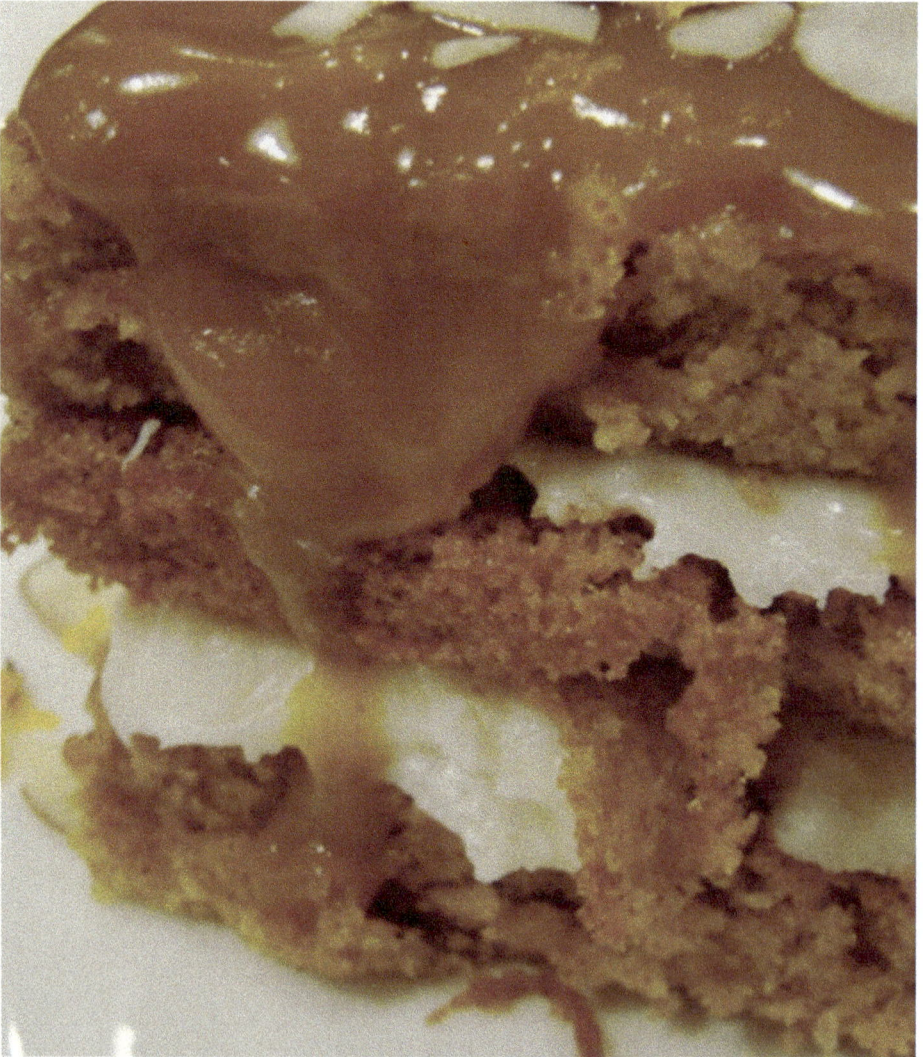

# Strawberry Sorbet

***Preparation Time:*** 5 minutes

**Cooking Time***: 4 Hours*

Servings: *4*

## Ingredients:

- 2 cups of Strawberries*
- 1 1/2 teaspoons of Spelt Flour
- 1/2 cup of Date Sugar
- 2 cups of Spring Water

## Directions:

- Add Date Sugar, Spring Water, and Spelt Flour to a medium pot and boil on low heat for about ten minutes. Mixture should thicken, like syrup.
- Remove the pot from the heat and allow it to cool.

- After cooling, add Blend Strawberry and mix gently.

- Put mixture in a container and freeze.

- Cut it into pieces, put the sorbet into a processor and blend until smooth.

- Put everything back in the container and leave in the refrigerator for at least four hours.

- Serve and enjoy your Strawberry Sorbet!

**_Nutrition:_** Calories: 198; Carbohydrates: 28 g

# Blueberry Muffins

***Preparation Time:*** 5 minutes

**Cooking Time***: 1 Hour*

Servings: *3*

## Ingredients:

- 1/2 cup of Blueberries

- 3/4 cup of Teff Flour

- 3/4 cup of Spelt Flour

- 1/3 cup of Agave Syrup

- 1/2 teaspoon of Pure Sea Salt

- 1 cup of Coconut Milk

- 1/4 cup of Sea Moss Gel (optional, check information)

- Grape Seed Oil

## Directions:

1. Preheat your oven to 365 degrees Fahrenheit.

2. Grease or line 6 standard muffin cups.

3. Add Teff, Spelt flour, Pure Sea Salt, Coconut Milk, Sea Moss Gel, and Agave Syrup to a large bowl. Mix them together.

4. Add Blueberries to the mixture and mix well.

5. Divide muffin batter among the 6 muffin cups.

6. Bake for 30 minutes until golden brown.

7. Serve and enjoy your Blueberry Muffins!

*__Nutrition:__* Calories: 65; Fat: 0.7 g; Carbohydrates: 12 g; Protein: 1.4 g; Fiber: 5 g

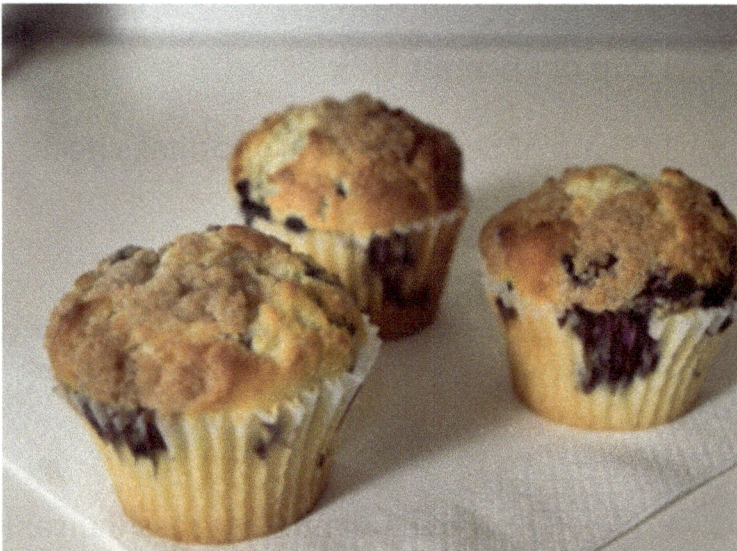

# Banana Strawberry Ice Cream

**_Preparation Time:_** 5 minutes

**Cooking Time**: _4 Hours_

Servings: _5_


## Ingredients:

- 1 cup of Strawberry*

- 5 quartered Baby Bananas*

- 1/2 Avocado, chopped

- 1 tablespoon of Agave Syrup

- 1/4 cup of Homemade Walnut Milk


## Directions:

1. Mix **Ingredients** into the blender and blend them well.

2. Taste. If it is too thick, add extra Milk or Agave Syrup if you want it sweeter.

3. Put in a container with a lid and allow to freeze for at least 5 to 6 hours.

1. Serve it and enjoy your Banana Strawberry Ice Cream!

**_Nutrition:_** Calories: 200; Fat: 0.5 g; Carbohydrates: 44 g

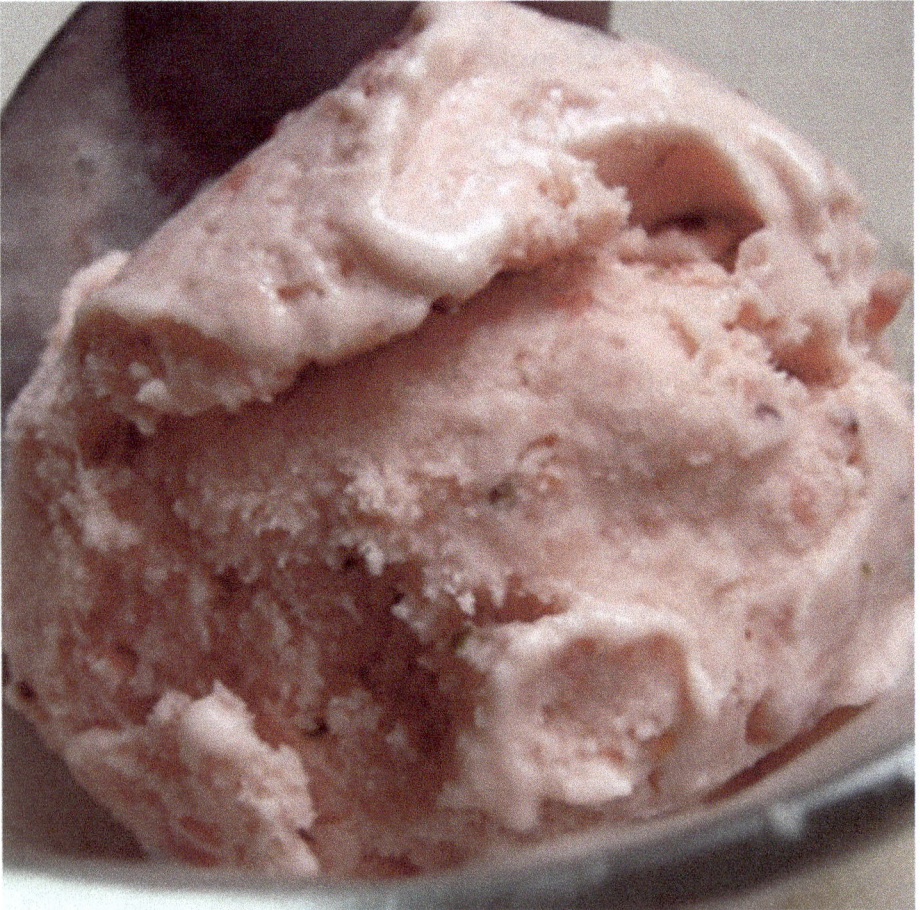

# Homemade Whipped Cream

**_Preparation Time:_** 5 minutes

**_Cooking Time_**: 10 Minutes

_Servings:_ 1 Cup

## Ingredients:

- 1 cup of Aquafaba

- 1/4 cup of Agave Syrup

## Directions:

1. Add Agave Syrup and Aquafaba into a bowl.

2. Mix at high speed around 5 minutes with a stand mixer or 10 to 15 minutes with a hand mixer.

3. Serve and enjoy your Homemade Whipped Cream!

***Nutrition:*** Calories: 21; Fat: 0g; Sodium: 0.3g; Carbohydrates: 5.3g; Fiber: 0g; Sugars: 4.7g; Protein: 0g

# Chocolate Crunch Bars

***Preparation Time:*** 5 minutes

**Cooking Time:** *5 minutes*

Servings: *4*

## Ingredients:

- 1 1/2 cups sugar-free chocolate chips
- 1 cup almond butter
- Stevia to taste
- 1/4 cup coconut oil
- 3 cups pecans, chopped

## Directions:

1. Layer an 8-inch baking pan with parchment paper.
2. Mix chocolate chips with butter, coconut oil, and sweetener in a bowl.

3. Melt it by heating in a microwave for 2 to 3 minutes until well mixed.

4. Stir in nuts and seeds. Mix gently.

5. Pour this batter carefully into the baking pan and spread evenly.

6. Refrigerate for 2 to 3 hours.

7. Slice and serve.

*__Nutrition:__* Calories 316; Total Fat 30.9 g; Saturated Fat 8.1 g; Cholesterol 0 mg; Total Carbs 8.3 g; Sugar 1.8 g; Fiber 3.8 g; Sodium 8 mg; Protein 6.4 g

# Homemade Protein Bar

**_Preparation Time:_** 5 minutes

**_Cooking Time_:** 10 minutes

Servings: _4_

## Ingredients:

- 1 cup nut butter
- 4 tablespoons coconut oil
- 2 scoops vanilla protein
- Stevia, to taste
- ½ teaspoon sea salt
- Optional Ingredients
- 1 teaspoon cinnamon

## Directions:

1. Mix coconut oil with butter, protein, stevia, and salt in a dish.
2. Stir in cinnamon and chocolate chip.

3. Press the mixture firmly and freeze until firm.

4. Cut the crust into small bars.

5. Serve and enjoy.

**Nutrition:** Calories 179; Total Fat 15.7 g; Saturated Fat 8 g; Cholesterol 0 mg; Total Carbs 4.8 g; Sugar 3.6 g; Fiber 0.8 g; Sodium 43 mg; Protein 5.6 g

# Shortbread Cookies

***Preparation Time:*** 10 minutes

***Cooking Time***: 70 minutes

Servings: *6*

## Ingredients:

- 2 1/2 cups almond flour

- 6 tablespoons nut butter

- 1/2 cup erythritol

- 1 teaspoon vanilla essence

## Directions:

1. Preheat your oven to 350 degrees F.

2. Layer a cookie sheet with parchment paper.

3. Beat butter with erythritol until fluffy.

4. Stir in vanilla essence and almond flour. Mix well until becomes crumbly.

5. Spoon out a tablespoon of cookie dough onto the cookie sheet.

6. Add more dough to make as many cookies.

7. Bake for 15 minutes until brown.

8. Serve.

**_Nutrition:_** Calories 288; Total Fat 25.3 g; Saturated Fat 6.7 g; Cholesterol 23 mg; Total Carbs 9.6 g; Sugar 0.1 g; Fiber 3.8 g; Sodium 74 mg; Potassium 3 mg; Protein 7.6 g

# Coconut Chip Cookies

***Preparation Time:*** 10 minutes

***Cooking Time***: 15 minutes

Servings: *4*

## Ingredients:

- 1 cup almond flour
- ½ cup cacao nibs
- ½ cup coconut flakes, unsweetened
- 1/3 cup erythritol
- ½ cup almond butter
- ¼ cup nut butter, melted
- ¼ cup almond milk
- Stevia, to taste
- ¼ teaspoon sea salt

## Directions:

1. Preheat your oven to 350 degrees F.

2. Layer a cookie sheet with parchment paper.

3. Add and then combine all the dry **Ingredients** in a glass bowl.

4. Whisk in butter, almond milk, vanilla essence, stevia, and almond butter.

5. Beat well then stir in dry mixture. Mix well.

6. Spoon out a tablespoon of cookie dough on the cookie sheet.

7. Add more dough to make as many as 16 cookies.

8. Flatten each cookie using your fingers.

9. Bake for 25 minutes until golden brown.

10. Let them sit for 15 minutes.

11. Serve.

**_Nutrition:_** Calories 192; Total Fat 17.44 g; Saturated Fat 11.5 g; Cholesterol 125 mg; Total Carbs 2.2 g; Sugar 1.4 g; Fiber 2.1 g; Sodium 135 mg; Protein 4.7 g

# Peanut Butter Bars

***Preparation Time:*** 10 minutes

***Cooking Time***: 10 minutes

Servings: 6

## Ingredients:

- 3/4 cup almond flour

- 2 oz. almond butter

- 1/4 cup Swerve

- 1/2 cup peanut butter

- 1/2 teaspoon vanilla

## Directions:

1. Combine all the Ingredients for bars.

2. Transfer this mixture to 6-inch small pan. Press it firmly.

3. Refrigerate for 30 minutes.

4. Slice and serve.

**_Nutrition:_** Calories 214; Total Fat 19 g; Saturated Fat 5.8 g; Cholesterol 15 mg; Total Carbs 6.5 g; Sugar 1.9 g; Fiber 2.1 g; Sodium 123 mg; Protein 6.5 g

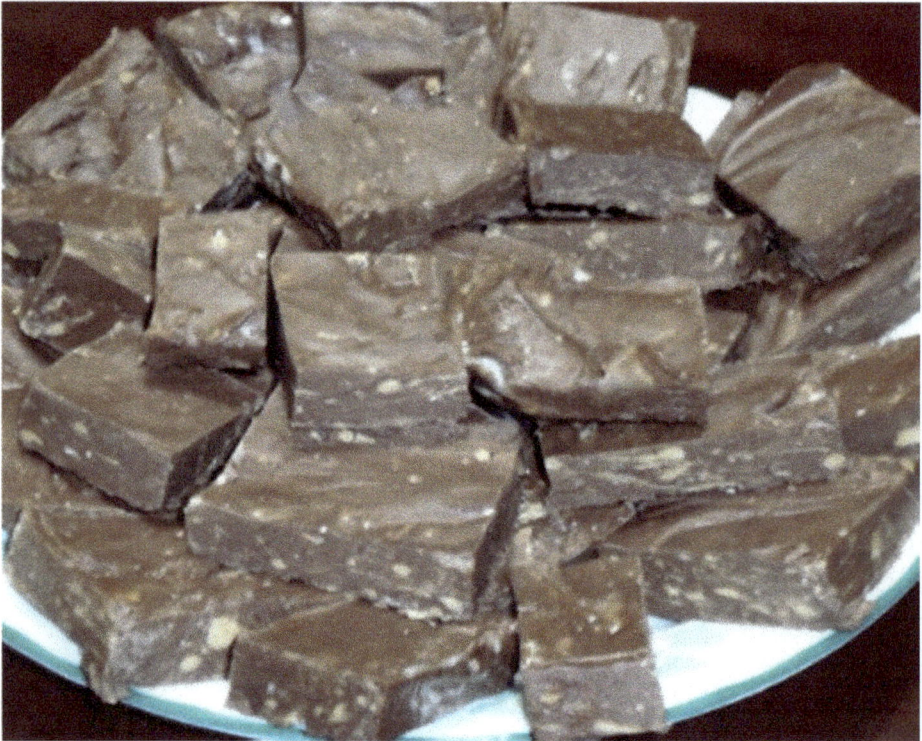

# Zucchini Bread Pancakes

*Preparation Time:* 15 minutes

*Cooking Time*: 35 minutes

*Servings:* 3

## Ingredients:

- Grapeseed oil, 1 tbsp.
- Chopped walnuts, .5 c
- Walnut milk, 2 c
- Shredded zucchini, 1 c
- Mashed burro banana, .25 c
- Date sugar, 2 tbsp.
- Kamut flour or spelt, 2 c

## Directions:

1. Place the date sugar and flour into a bowl. Whisk together.

2. Add in the mashed banana and walnut milk. Stir until combined. Remember to scrape the bowl to get all the dry mixture. Add in walnuts and zucchini. Stir well until combined.

3. Place the grapeseed oil onto a griddle and warm.

4. Pour .25 cup batter on the hot griddle. Leave it along until bubbles begin forming on to surface. Carefully turn over the pancake and cook another four minutes until cooked through.

5. Place the pancakes onto a **Serving** plate and enjoy with some agave syrup.

**_Nutrition:_** Calories: 246; Carbohydrates: 49.2 g; Fiber: 4.6 g; Protein: 7.8

# Flourless Chocolate Cake

***Preparation Time:*** 10 minutes

***Cooking Time***: 45 minutes

Servings: 6

## Ingredients:

- 1/2 Cup of stevia

- 12 Ounces of unsweetened baking chocolate

- 2/3 Cup of ghee

- 1/3 Cup of warm water

- ¼ Teaspoon of salt

- 4 Large pastured eggs

- 2 Cups of boiling water

## Directions:

1. Line the bottom of a 9-inch pan of a spring form with a parchment paper.

2. Heat the water in a small pot; then add the salt and the stevia over the water until wait until the mixture becomes completely dissolved.

3. Melt the baking chocolate into a double boiler or simply microwave it for about 30 seconds.

4. Mix the melted chocolate and the butter in a large bowl with an electric mixer.

5. Beat in your hot mixture; then crack in the egg and whisk after adding each of the eggs.

6. Pour the obtained mixture into your prepared spring form tray.

7. Wrap the spring form tray with a foil paper.

8. Place the spring form tray in a large cake tray and add boiling water right to the outside; make sure the depth doesn't exceed 1 inch.

9. Bake the cake into the water bath for about 45 minutes at a temperature of about 350 F.

10. Remove the tray from the boiling water and transfer to a wire to cool.

11.  Let the cake chill for an overnight in the refrigerator.

12.  Serve and enjoy your delicious cake!

**_Nutrition:_** Calories: 295; Fat: 26g; Carbohydrates: 6g; Fiber: 4g; Protein: 8g

# Raspberry Cake With White Chocolate Sauce

***Preparation Time:*** 15 minutes

***Cooking Time***: 60 minutes

Servings: 6

## Ingredients:

- 5 Ounces of melted cacao butter

- 2 Ounces of grass-fed ghee

- 1/2 Cup of coconut cream

- 1 Cup of green banana flour

- 3 Teaspoons of pure vanilla

- 4 Large eggs

- 1/2 Cup of as Lakanto Monk Fruit

- 1 Teaspoon of baking powder

- 2 Teaspoons of apple cider vinegar

- 2 Cup of raspberries

For the white chocolate sauce:

- 3 and 1/2 ounces of cacao butter

- 1/2 Cup of coconut cream

- 2 Teaspoons of pure vanilla extract

- 1 Pinch of salt

## Directions:

1. Preheat your oven to a temperature of about 280 degrees Fahrenheit.

2. Combine the green banana flour with the pure vanilla extract, the baking powder, the coconut cream, the eggs, the cider vinegar and the monk fruit and mix very well.

3. Leave the raspberries aside and line a cake loaf tin with a baking paper.

4. Pour in the batter into the baking tray and scatter the raspberries over the top of the cake.

5. Place the tray in your oven and bake it for about 60 minutes; in the meantime, prepare the sauce by

**Directions** for sauce:

6. Combine the cacao cream, the vanilla extract, the cacao butter and the salt in a saucepan over a low heat

7. Mix all your **Ingredients** with a fork to make sure the cacao butter mixes very well with the cream.

8. Remove from the heat and set aside to cool a little bit; but don't let it harden.

9. Drizzle with the chocolate sauce.

10. Scatter the cake with more raspberries.

11. Slice your cake; then serve and enjoy it!

**_Nutrition:_** Calories: 323; Fat: 31.5g; Carbohydrates: 9.9g; Fiber: 4g; Protein: 5g

# Ketogenic Lava Cake

**Preparation Time:** *10 minutes*

**_Cooking Time_**: 10 minutes

Servings: *2*

## Ingredients:

- 2 Oz of dark chocolate; you should at least use chocolate of 85% cocoa solids
- 1 Tablespoon of super-fine almond flour
- 2 Oz of unsalted almond butter
- 2 Large eggs

## Directions:

1. Heat your oven to a temperature of about 350 Fahrenheit.
2. Grease 2 heat proof ramekins with almond butter.

3. Now, melt the chocolate and the almond butter and stir very well.

4. Beat the eggs very well with a mixer.

5. Add the eggs to the chocolate and the butter mixture and mix very well with almond flour and the swerve; then stir.

6. Pour the dough into 2 ramekins.

7. Bake for about 9 to 10 minutes.

8. Turn the cakes over plates and serve with pomegranate seeds!

**Nutrition:** Calories: 459; Fat: 39g; Carbohydrates: 3.5g; Fiber: 0.8g; Protein: 11.7g

# Ketogenic Cheese Cake

**Preparation Time:** *15 minutes*

**_Cooking Time_**: 50 minutes

Servings: 6

## Ingredients:

For the Almond Flour Cheesecake Crust:

- 2 Cups of Blanched almond flour

- 1/3 Cup of almond Butter

- 3 Tablespoons of Erythritol (powdered or granular)

- 1 Teaspoon of Vanilla extract

For the Keto Cheesecake Filling:

- 32 Oz of softened Cream cheese

- 1 and ¼ cups of powdered erythritol

- 3 Large Eggs

- 1 Tablespoon of Lemon juice

- 1 Teaspoon of Vanilla extract

## Directions:

1. Preheat your oven to a temperature of about 350 degrees F.

2. Grease a spring form pan of 9" with cooking spray or just line its bottom with a parchment paper.

3. In order to make the cheesecake rust, stir in the melted butter, the almond flour, the vanilla extract and the erythritol in a large bowl.

4. The dough will get will be a bit crumbly; so, press it into the bottom of your prepared tray.

5. Bake for about 12 minutes; then let cool for about 10 minutes.

6. In the meantime, beat the softened cream cheese and the powdered sweetener at a low speed until it becomes smooth.

7. Crack in the eggs and beat them in at a low to medium speed until it becomes fluffy. Make sure to add one a time.

8. Add in the lemon juice and the vanilla extract and mix at a low to medium speed with a mixer.

9. Pour your filling into your pan right on top of the crust. You can use a spatula to smooth the top of the cake.

10. Bake for about 45 to 50 minutes.

11. Remove the baked cheesecake from your oven and run a knife around its edge.

12. Let the cake cool for about 4 hours in the refrigerator.

13. Serve and enjoy your delicious cheese cake!


**_Nutrition:_** Calories: 325; Fat: 29g; Carbohydrates: 6g; Fiber: 1g; Protein: 7g

# Cake with Whipped Cream Icing

**Preparation Time:** *20 minutes*

***Cooking Time***: 25 minutes

Servings: *7*

## Ingredients:

- ¾ Cup Coconut flour
- ¾ Cup of Swerve Sweetener
- 1/2 Cup of Cocoa powder
- 2 Teaspoons of Baking powder
- 6 Large Eggs
- 2/3 Cup of Heavy Whipping Cream
- 1/2 Cup of Melted almond Butter

For the whipped Cream Icing:

- 1 Cup of Heavy Whipping Cream
- ¼ Cup of Swerve Sweetener
- 1 Teaspoon of Vanilla extract

- 1/3 Cup of Sifted Cocoa Powder

## Directions:

1. Pre-heat your oven to a temperature of about 350 F.

2. Grease an 8x8 cake tray with cooking spray.

3. Add the coconut flour, the Swerve sweetener; the cocoa powder, the baking powder, the eggs, the melted butter; and combine very well with an electric or a hand mixer.

4. Pour your batter into the cake tray and bake for about 25 minutes.

5. Remove the cake tray from the oven and let cool for about 5 minutes.

For the Icing

6. Whip the cream until it becomes fluffy; then add in the Swerve, the vanilla and the cocoa powder.

7. Add the Swerve, the vanilla and the cocoa powder; then continue mixing until your **Ingredients** are very well combined.

8. Frost your baked cake with the icing; then slice it; serve and enjoy your delicious cake!


_**Nutrition:**_ Calories: 357, Fat: 33g; Carbohydrates: 11g; Fiber: 2g; Protein: 8g

# Walnut-Fruit Cake

**Preparation Time:** *15 minutes*

***Cooking Time***: 20 minutes

Servings: *6*

## Ingredients:

- 1/2 Cup of almond butter (softened)
- ¼ Cup of so Nourished granulated erythritol
- 1 Tablespoon of ground cinnamon
- 1/2 Teaspoon of ground nutmeg
- ¼ Teaspoon of ground cloves
- 4 Large pastured eggs
- 1 Teaspoon of vanilla extract
- 1/2 Teaspoon of almond extract
- 2 Cups of almond flour
- 1/2 Cup of chopped walnuts
- ¼ Cup of dried of unsweetened cranberries

- ¼ Cup of seedless raisins

## Directions:

1. Preheat your oven to a temperature of about 350 F and grease an 8-inch baking tin of round shape with coconut oil.

2. Beat the granulated erythritol on a high speed until it becomes fluffy.

3. Add the cinnamon, the nutmeg, and the cloves; then blend your **Ingredients** until they become smooth.

4. Crack in the eggs and beat very well by adding one at a time, plus the almond extract and the vanilla.

5. Whisk in the almond flour until it forms a smooth batter then fold in the nuts and the fruit.

6. Spread your mixture into your prepared baking pan and bake it for about 20 minutes.

7. Remove the cake from the oven and let cool for about 5 minutes.

8. Dust the cake with the powdered erythritol.

9. Serve and enjoy your cake!

**_Nutrition:_** Calories: 250; Fat: 11g; Carbohydrates: 12g; Fiber: 2g; Protein: 7g

# Ginger Cake

**Preparation Time:** *15 minutes*

*Cooking Time*: 20 minutes

Servings: *9*

## Ingredients:

- 1/2 Tablespoon of unsalted almond butter to grease the pan
- 4 Large eggs
- ¼ Cup coconut milk
- 2 Tablespoons of unsalted almond butter
- 1 and 1/2 teaspoons of stevia
- 1 Tablespoon of ground cinnamon
- 1 Tablespoon of natural unweeded cocoa powder
- 1 Tablespoon of fresh ground ginger
- 1/2 Teaspoon of kosher salt
- 1 and 1/2 cups of blanched almond flour

- 1/2 Teaspoon of baking soda

## Directions:

1. Preheat your oven to a temperature of 325 F.

2. Grease a glass baking tray of about 8X8 inches generously with almond butter.

3. In a large bowl, whisk all together the coconut milk, the eggs, the melted almond butter, the stevia, the cinnamon, the cocoa powder, the ginger and the kosher salt.

4. Whisk in the almond flour, then the baking soda and mix very well.

5. Pour the batter into the prepared pan and bake for about 20 to 25 minutes.

6. Let the cake cool for about 5 minutes; then slice; serve and enjoy your delicious cake.

*Nutrition:* Calories: 175; Fat: 15g ; Carbohydrates: 5g; Fiber: 1.9g; Protein: 5g

# Ketogenic Orange Cake

**Preparation Time:** *10 minutes*

***Cooking Time***: 50minutes

Servings: *8*

## Ingredients:

- 2 and 1/2 cups of almond flour

- 2 Unwaxed washed oranges

- 5 Large separated eggs

- 1 Teaspoon of baking powder

- 2 Teaspoons of orange extract

- 1 Teaspoon of vanilla bean powder

- 6 Seeds of cardamom pods crushed

- 16 drops of liquid stevia; about 3 teaspoons

- 1 Handful of flaked almonds to decorate

## Directions:

1. Preheat your oven to a temperature of about 350 Fahrenheit.

2. Line a rectangular bread baking tray with a parchment paper.

3. Place the oranges into a pan filled with cold water and cover it with a lid.

4. Bring the saucepan to a boil, then let simmer for about 1 hour and make sure the oranges are totally submerged.

5. Make sure the oranges are always submerged to remove any taste of bitterness.

6. Cut the oranges into halves; then remove any seeds; and drain the water and set the oranges aside to cool down.

7. Cut the oranges in half and remove any seeds, then puree it with a blender or a food processor.

8. Separate the eggs; then whisk the egg whites until you see stiff peaks forming.

9. Add all your **Ingredients** except for the egg whites to the orange mixture and add in the egg whites; then mix.

10.    Pour the batter into the cake tin and sprinkle with the flaked almonds right on top.

11.    Bake your cake for about 50 minutes.

12.    Remove the cake from the oven and set aside to cool for 5 minutes.

13.  Slice your cake; then serve and enjoy its incredible taste!

*__Nutrition:__* Calories: 164; Fat: 12g; Carbohydrates: 7.1; Fiber: 2.7g; Protein: 10.9g

# Lemon Cake

**Preparation Time:** *20 minutes*

***Cooking Time***: 20minutes

Servings: *6*

## Ingredients:

- 2 Medium lemons
- 4 Large eggs
- 2 Tablespoons of almond butter
- 2 Tablespoons of avocado oil
- 1/3 cup of coconut flour
- 4-5 tablespoons of honey (or another sweetener of your choice)
- 1/2 tablespoon of baking soda

## Directions:

1. Preheat your oven to a temperature of about 350 F.

2. Crack the eggs in a large bowl and set two egg whites aside.

3. Whisk the 2 whites of eggs with the egg yolks, the honey, the oil, the almond butter, the lemon zest and the juice and whisk very well together.

4. Combine the baking soda with the coconut flour and gradually add this dry mixture to the wet **Ingredients** and keep whisking for a couple of minutes.

5. Beat the two eggs with a hand mixer and beat the egg into foam.

6. Add the white egg foam gradually to the mixture with a silicone spatula.

7. Transfer your obtained batter to tray covered with a baking paper.

8. Bake your cake for about 20 to 22 minutes.

9. Let the cake cool for 5 minutes; then slice your cake.

10. Serve and enjoy your delicious cake!

***Nutrition:*** Calories: 164; Fat: 12g; Carbohydrates: 7.1;
Fiber: 2.7g; Protein: 10.9g

# Cinnamon Cake

***Preparation Time:*** 15 minutes

***Cooking Time***: 35minutes

Servings: *6*

## Ingredients:

For the Cinnamon Filling:

- 3 Tablespoons of Swerve Sweetener

- 2 Teaspoons of ground cinnamon

For the Cake:

- 3 Cups of almond flour

- ¾ Cup of Swerve Sweetener

- ¼ Cup of unflavored whey protein powder

- 2 Teaspoon of baking powder

- 1/2 Teaspoon of salt

- 3 large pastured eggs

- 1/2 Cup of melted coconut oil

- 1/2 Teaspoon of vanilla extract

- 1/2 Cup of almond milk

- 1 Tablespoon of melted coconut oil

For the cream cheese Frosting:

- 3 Tablespoons of softened cream cheese

- 2 Tablespoons of powdered Swerve Sweetener

- 1 Tablespoon of coconut heavy whipping cream

- 1/2 Teaspoon of vanilla extract

## Directions:

1. Preheat your oven to a temperature of about 325 F and grease a baking tray of 8x8 inch.

2. For the filling, mix the Swerve and the cinnamon in a mixing bowl and mix very well; then set it aside.

3. For the preparation of the cake; whisk all together the almond flour, the sweetener, the

protein powder, the baking powder, and the salt in a mixing bowl.

4. Add in the eggs, the melted coconut oil and the vanilla extract and mix very well.

5. Add in the almond milk and keep stirring until your **Ingredients** are very well combined.

6. Spread about half of the batter in the prepared pan; then sprinkle with about two thirds of the filling mixture.

7. Spread the remaining mixture of the batter over the filling and smooth it with a spatula.

8. Bake for about 35 minutes in the oven.

9. Brush with the melted coconut oil and sprinkle with the remaining cinnamon filling.

10.   Prepare the frosting by beating the cream cheese, the powdered erythritol, the cream and the vanilla extract in a mixing bowl until it becomes smooth.

11.   Drizzle frost over the cooled cake.

12. Slice the cake; then serve and enjoy your cake!

**_Nutrition:_** Calories: 222; Fat: 19.2g; Carbohydrates: 5.4g; Fiber: 1.5g; Protein: 7.3g

# Banana Nut Muffins

*__Preparation Time:__* 5 minutes

*__Cooking Time__*: 1 Hour

*__Servings:__* 6

*__Ingredients:__*

Dry **Ingredients:**

- 1 1/2 cups of Spell or Teff Flour

- 1/2 teaspoon of Pure Sea Salt

- 3/4 cup of Date Syrup

Wet **Ingredients:**

- 2 medium Blend Burro Bananas

- ¼ cup of Grape Seed Oil

- ¾ cup of Homemade Walnut Milk (see recipe)*

- 1 tablespoon of Key Lime Juice

Filling **Ingredients:**

- ½ cup of chopped Walnuts (plus extra for decorating)

- 1 chopped Burro Banana

## Directions:

1. Preheat your oven to 400 degrees Fahrenheit.

2. Take a muffin tray and grease 12 cups or line with cupcake liners.

3. Put all dry **Ingredients** in a large bowl and mix them thoroughly.

4. Add all wet **Ingredients** to a separate, smaller bowl and mix well with Blend Bananas.

5. Mix **Ingredients** from the two bowls in one large container. Be careful not to over mix.

6. Add the filling **Ingredients** and fold in gently.

7. Pour muffin batter into the 12 prepared muffin cups and garnish with a couple Walnuts.

8. Bake it for 22 to 26 minutes until golden brown.

9. Allow to cool for 10 minutes.

10. Serve and enjoy your Banana Nut Muffins!

***Nutrition:*** Calories: 150; Fat: 10 g; Carbohydrates: 30 g; Protein: 2.4 g; Fiber: 2 g

# Mango Nut Cheesecake

**_Cooking Time_**: 4 Hour 30 Minutes

**_Servings:_** 8 Servings

## **_Ingredients:_**

Filling:

- 2 cups of Brazil Nuts

- 5 to 6 Dates

- 1 tablespoon of Sea Moss Gel (check information)

- 1/4 cup of Agave Syrup

- 1/4 teaspoon of Pure Sea Salt

- 2 tablespoons of Lime Juice

- 1 1/2 cups of Homemade Walnut Milk (see recipe)*

Crust:

- 1 1/2 cups of quartered Dates

- 1/4 cup of Agave Syrup

- 1 1/2 cups of Coconut Flakes

- 1/4 teaspoon of Pure Sea Salt

Toppings:

- Sliced Mango

- Sliced Strawberries

## Directions:

1. Put all crust **Ingredients** , in a food processor and blend for 30 seconds.

2. With parchment paper, cover a baking form and spread out the blended crust **Ingredients** .

3. Put sliced Mango across the crust and freeze for 10 minutes.

4. Mix all filling **Ingredients** , using a blender until it becomes smooth

5. Pour the filling above the crust, cover with foil or parchment paper and let it stand for about 3 to 4 hours in the refrigerator.

6. Take out from the baking form and garnish with toppings.

7. Serve and enjoy your Mango Nut Cheesecake!

# Blackberry Jam

*Preparation Time:* 5 minutes

*Cooking Time*: 4 Hour 30 Minutes

*Servings:* 1 Cup

## Ingredients:

- 3/4 cup of Blackberries

- 1 tablespoon of Key Lime Juice

- 3 tablespoons of Agave Syrup

- ¼ cup of Sea Moss Gel + extra 2 tablespoons (check information)

## Directions:

1. Put rinsed Blackberries into a medium pot and cook on medium heat.

2. Stir Blackberries until liquid appears.

3. Once berries soften, use your immersion blender to chop up any large pieces. If you

don't have a blender, put the mixture in a food processor, mix it well, then return to the pot.

4. Add Sea Moss Gel, Key Lime Juice and Agave Syrup to the blended mixture. Boil on medium heat and stir well until it becomes thick.

5. Remove from the heat and leave it to cool for 10 minutes.

6. Serve it with bread pieces or the Flatbread (see recipe).

7. Enjoy your Blackberry Jam!

**Nutrition:** Calories: 43; Fat: 0.5 g; Carbohydrates: 13 g

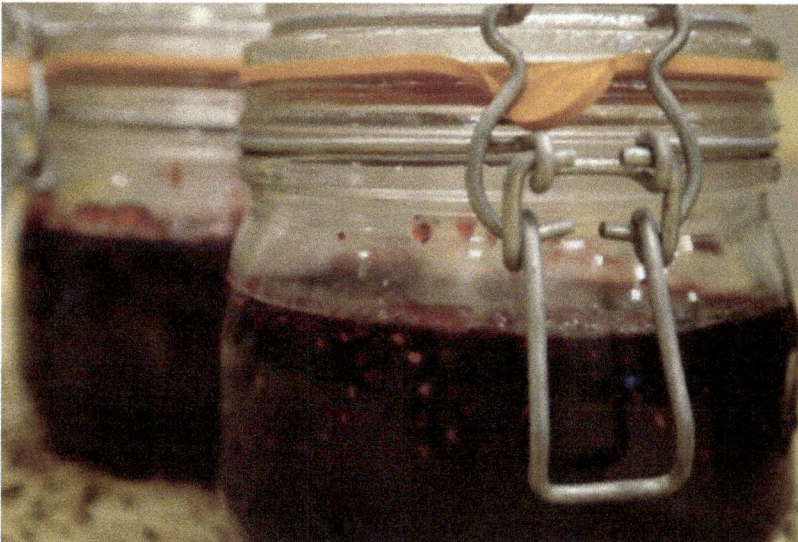

# Blackberry Bars

***Preparation Time:*** 5 minutes

***Cooking Time***: 1 Hour 20 Minutes

Servings: *4*

## Ingredients:

- 3 Burro Bananas or 4 Baby Bananas
- 1 cup of Spelt Flour
- 2 cups of Quinoa Flakes
- 1/4 cup of Agave Syrup
- 1/4 teaspoon of Pure Sea Salt
- 1/2 cup of Grape Seed Oil
- 1 cup of prepared Blackberry Jam

## Directions:

1. Preheat your oven to 350 degrees Fahrenheit.
2. Remove skin of Bananas and mash with a fork in a large bowl.

3. Combine Agave Syrup and Grape Seed Oil with the Blend and mix well.

4. Add Spelt Flour and Quinoa Flakes. Knead the dough until it becomes sticky to your fingers.

5. Cover a 9x9-inch baking pan with parchment paper.

6. Take 2/3 of the dough and smooth it out over the parchment pan with your fingers.

7. Spread Blackberry Jam over the dough.

8. Crumble the remainder dough and sprinkle on the top.

9. Bake for 20 minutes.

10. Remove from the oven and let it cool for at 10 to 15 minutes.

11. Cut into small pieces.

12. Serve and enjoy your Blackberry Bars!

**_Nutrition:_** Calories: 43; Fat: 0.5 g; Carbohydrates: 10 g; Protein: 1.4 g; Fiber: 5 g

# Detox Berry Smoothie

**_Preparation Time:_** 15 minutes

**Cooking Time**: *0*

*Servings:* 1

## Ingredients:

- Spring water

- 1/4 avocado, pitted

- One medium burro banana

- One Seville orange

- Two cups of fresh lettuce

- One tablespoon of hemp seeds

- One cup of berries (blueberries or an aggregate of blueberries, strawberries, and raspberries)

## Directions:

1. Add the spring water to your blender.

2. Put the fruits and vegies right inside the blender.

3. *Blend all **Ingredients** till smooth.*

**<u>Nutrition:</u>** Calories: 202.4; Fat: 4.5g ; Carbohydrates: 32.9g ; Protein: 13.3g

# Dandelion Avocado Smoothie

***Preparation Time:*** 15 minutes

**Cooking Time**: *0*

Servings: *1*

## Ingredients:

- One cup of Dandelion

- One Orange (juiced)

- Coconut water

- One Avocado

- One key lime (juice)

## *Directions:*

1. In a high-speed blender until smooth, blend **Ingredients**.

***Nutrition:*** Calories: 160; Fat: 15 g; Carbohydrates: 9 g; Protein: 2 g

# Amaranth Greens and Avocado Smoothie

**_Preparation Time:_** 15 minutes

**Cooking Time**: 0

Servings: 1

## Ingredients:

- One key lime (juice).

- Two sliced apples (seeded).

- Half avocado.

- Two cupsful of amaranth greens.

- Two cupsful of watercress.

- One cupful of water.

## _Directions:_

1. Add the whole recipes together and transfer them into the blender. Blend thoroughly until smooth.

***Nutrition:*** Calories: 160; Fat: 15 g; Carbohydrates: 9 g; Protein: 2 g

# Lettuce, Orange and Banana Smoothie

**_Preparation Time:_** 15 minutes

**Cooking Time**_: 0_

_Servings:_ 1

**_Ingredients:_**

- One and a half cupsful of fresh lettuce.

- One large banana.

- One cup of mixed berries of your choice.

- One juiced orange.

**Directions:**

1. First, add the orange juice to your blender.

2. Add the remaining recipes and blend thoroughly.

3. Enjoy the rest of your day.

**_Nutrition:_** Calories: 252.1; Protein: 4.1 g

# Delicious Elderberry Smoothie

*Preparation Time:* 15 minutes

**Cooking Time***: 0*

*Servings:* 1

## Ingredients:

- One cupful of Elderberry
- One cupful of Cucumber
- One large apple
- A quarter cupful of water

## Directions:

1. Add the whole recipes together into a blender. Grind very well until they are uniformly smooth and enjoy.

*Nutrition:* Calories: 106; Carbohydrates: 26.68

# Peaches Zucchini Smoothie

***Preparation Time:*** 15 minutes

**Cooking Time***: 0*

*Servings:* 1

***Ingredients:***

- A half cupful of squash.

- A half cupful of peaches.

- A quarter cupful of coconut water.

- A half cupful of Zucchini.

## Directions:

1. Add the whole recipes together into a blender and blend until smooth and serve.

***Nutrition:*** 55 Calories; 0g Fat; 2g Of Protein; 10mg Sodium; 14 G Carbohydrate; 2g Of Fiber

# Ginger Orange and Strawberry Smoothie

**Preparation Time:** 15 minutes

**Cooking Time**: 0

Servings: 1

## Ingredients:

- One cup of strawberry.

- One large orange (juice)

- One large banana.

- Quarter small sized ginger (peeled and sliced).

## *Directions:*

2. Transfer the orange juice to a clean blender.

3. Add the remaining recipes and blend thoroughly until smooth.

4. Enjoy. Wow! You have ended the 9th day of your weight loss and detox journey.

***Nutrition:*** 32 Calories; 0.3g Fat; 2g Of Protein; 10mg Sodium; 14g Carbohydrate; Water; 2g Of Fiber.

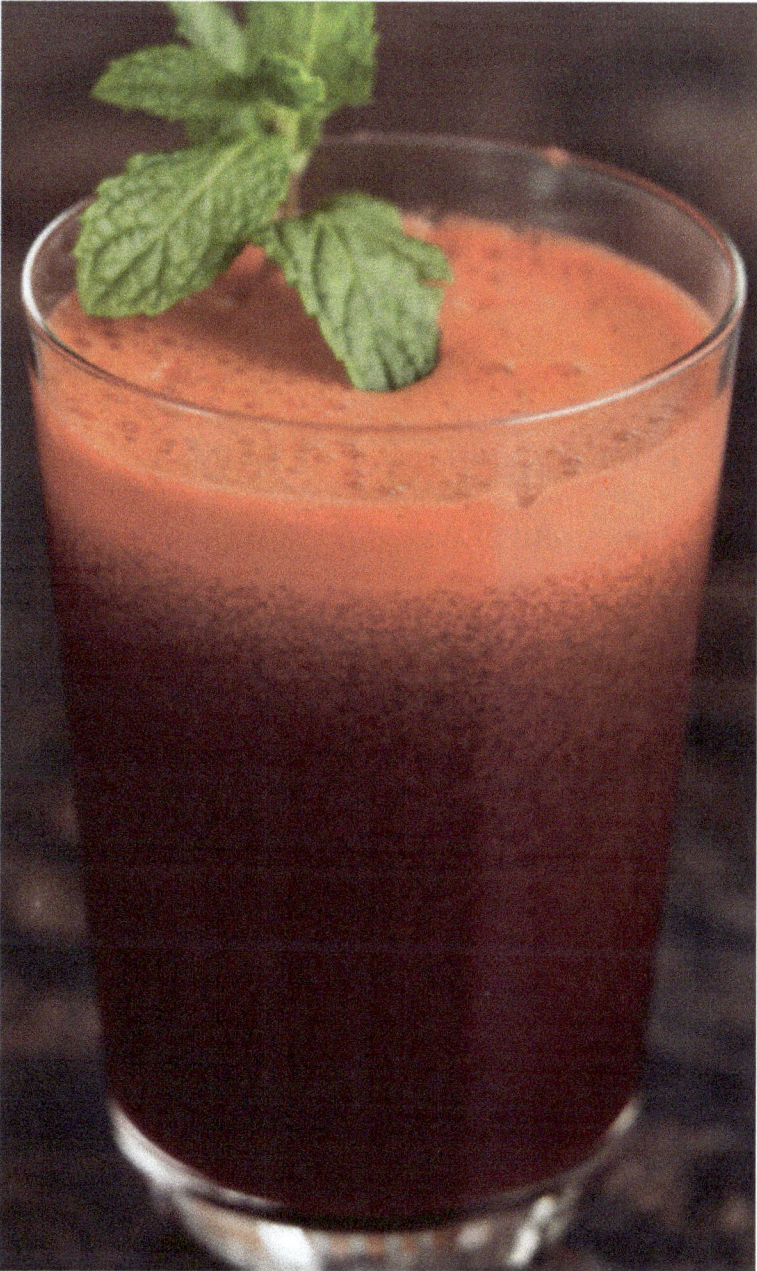

# Kale Parsley and Chia Seeds Detox Smoothie

***Preparation Time:*** 15 minutes

**Cooking Time***: 0*

*Servings:* 1

## *Ingredients:*

- Three tbsp. chia seeds (grounded).

- One cupful of water.

- One sliced banana.

- One pear (chopped).

- One cupful of organic kale.

- One cupful of parsley.

- Two tbsp. of lemon juice.

- A dash of cinnamon.

### Directions:

1. Add the whole recipes together into a blender and pour the water before blending. Blend at high speed until smooth and enjoy. You may or may not place it in the refrigerator depending on how hot or cold the weather appears.

**Nutrition:** 75 calories; 1g fat; 5g protein; 10g fiber

# Watermelon Limenade

**_Preparation Time:_** 5 Minutes

**_Cooking Time_**: 0 minutes

Servings: 6

When it comes to refreshing summertime drinks, lemonade is always near the top of the list. This Watermelon "Limenade" is perfect for using up leftover watermelon or for those early fall days when stores and farmers are almost giving them away. You can also substitute 4 cups of ice for the cold water to create a delicious summertime slushy.

## _Ingredients:_

- 4 cups diced watermelon
- 4 cups cold water
- 2 tablespoons freshly squeezed lemon juice
- 1 tablespoon freshly squeezed lime juice

## Directions:

1. In a blender, combine the watermelon, water, lemon juice, and lime juice, and blend for 1 minute.

2. Strain the contents through a fine-mesh sieve or nut-milk bag. Serve chilled. Store in the refrigerator for up to 3 days.

**SERVING** TIP: Slice up a few lemon or lime wedges to serve with your Watermelon Limenade, or top it with a few fresh mint leaves to give it an extra-crisp, minty flavor.

***Nutrition:*** Calories: 60

# Bubbly Orange Soda

*__Preparation Time:__* 5 Minutes

*__Cooking Time__*: 0 minutes

Servings: *4*

Soda can be one of the toughest things to give up when you first adopt a WFPB diet. That's partially because refined sugars and caffeine are addictive, but it can also be because carbonated beverages are fun to drink! With sweetness from the orange juice and bubbliness from the carbonated water, this orange "soda" is perfect for assisting in the transition from SAD to WFPB.

## Ingredients:

- 4 cups carbonated water

- 2 cups pulp-free orange juice (4 oranges, freshly squeezed and strained)

## Directions:

1. For each serving, pour 2 parts carbonated water and 1-part orange juice over ice right before serving.

2. Stir and enjoy.

**SERVING** TIP: This recipe is best made right before drinking. The amount of fizz in the carbonated water will decrease the longer it's open, so if you're going to make it ahead of time, make sure it's stored in an airtight, refrigerator-safe container.

*__Nutrition__:* Calories: 56

# Creamy Cashew Milk

*Preparation Time:* 5 Minutes

*Cooking Time*: 0 minutes

Servings: *8*

Learning how to make your own plant-based milks can be one of the best ways to save money and ditch dairy for good. This is one of the easiest milk recipes to master, and if you have a high-speed blender, you can skip the straining step and go straight to a refrigerator-safe container. Large mason jars work great for storing plant-based milk, as they allow you to give a quick shake before each use.

## Ingredients:

- 4 cups water
- ¼ cup raw cashews, soaked overnight

## Directions:

1. In a blender, blend the water and cashews on high speed for 2 minutes.

2. Strain with a nut-milk bag or cheesecloth, then store in the refrigerator for up to 5 days.

VARIATION TIP: This recipe makes unsweetened cashew milk that can be used in savory and sweet dishes. For a creamier version to put in your coffee, cut the amount of water in half. For a sweeter version, add 1 to 2 tablespoons maple syrup and 1 teaspoon vanilla extract before blending.

*__Nutrition__:* Calories: 18

# Homemade Oat Milk

*Preparation Time:* 5 Minutes

*Cooking Time*: 0 minutes

Servings: *8*

Oat milk is a fantastic option if you need a nut-free milk or just want an extremely inexpensive plant-based milk. Making a half-gallon jar at home costs a fraction of the price of other plant-based or dairy milks. Oat milk can be used in both savory and sweet dishes.

## Ingredients:

- 1 cup rolled oats
- 4 cups water

## Directions:

1. Put the oats in a medium bowl, and cover with cold water. Soak for 15 minutes, then drain and rinse the oats.

2.  Pour the cold water and the soaked oats into a blender. Blend for 60 to 90 seconds, or just until the mixture is a creamy white color throughout. (Blending any further may over blend the oats, resulting in a gummy milk.)

3.  Strain through a nut-milk bag or colander, then store in the refrigerator for up to 5 days.

**_Nutrition_**: Calories: 39

# Lucky Mint Smoothie

***Preparation Time:*** 5 Minutes

***Cooking Time***: 0 minutes

Servings: *2*

As spring approaches and mint begins to take over the garden once again, "Irish"-themed green shakes begin to pop up as well. In contrast to the traditionally high-fat, sugary shakes, this smoothie is a wonderful option for sunny spring days. So next time you want to sip on something cool and minty, do so with a health-promoting Lucky Mint Smoothie.

## Ingredients:

- 2 cups plant-based milk (here or here)

- 2 frozen bananas, halved

- 1 tablespoon fresh mint leaves or ¼ teaspoon peppermint extract

- 1 teaspoon vanilla extract

## Directions:

1. In a blender, combine the milk, bananas, mint, and vanilla. Blend on high for 1 to 2 minutes, or until the contents reach a smooth and creamy consistency, and serve.

2.

VARIATION TIP: If you like to sneak greens into smoothies, add a cup or two of spinach to boost the health benefits of this smoothie and give it an even greener appearance.

**Nutrition:** Calories: 152

# Paradise Island Smoothie

***Preparation Time:*** 5 Minutes

***Cooking Time***: 0 minutes

Servings: *2*

## Ingredients:

- 2 cups plant-based milk (here or here)
- 1 frozen banana
- ½ cup frozen mango chunks
- ½ cup frozen pineapple chunks
- 1 teaspoon vanilla extract

## Directions:

1. In a blender, combine the milk, banana, mango, pineapple, and vanilla. Blend on high for 1 to 2 minutes, or until the contents reach a smooth and creamy consistency, and serve.

LEFTOVER TIP: If you have any leftover smoothie, you can put it in a jar with some rolled oats and allow the mixture to soak in the refrigerator overnight to create a tropical version of overnight oats.

***Nutrition:*** Calories: 176

# Apple Pie Smoothie

***Preparation Time:*** 5 Minutes

***Cooking Time***: 0 minutes

Servings: *2*

This smoothie is great for a quick breakfast or a cool dessert. Its combination of sweet apples and warming cinnamon is sure to win over children and adults alike. If the holidays find you in a warm area, this smoothie may just be the cool treat you've been looking for to take the place of pie at dessert time.

## Ingredients:

- 2 sweet crisp apples, cut into 1-inch cubes
- 2 cups plant-based milk (here or here)
- 1 cup ice
- 1 tablespoon maple syrup
- 1 teaspoon ground cinnamon

- 1 teaspoon vanilla extract

## Directions:

1. In a blender, combine the apples, milk, ice, maple syrup, cinnamon, and vanilla. Blend on high for 1 to 2 minutes, or until the contents reach a smooth and creamy consistency, and serve.

VARIATION TIP: You can also use this recipe for making overnight oatmeal. Blend your smoothie, mix it with 2 cups rolled oats, and refrigerate overnight for a premade breakfast for two.

*Nutrition:* Calories: 198

# Choco-Nut Milkshake

***Preparation Time:*** 10 minutes

**Cooking Time***: 0 minute*

**Serving***: 2*

## Ingredients:

- 2 cups unsweetened coconut, almond
- 1 banana, sliced and frozen
- ¼ cup unsweetened coconut flakes
- 1 cup ice cubes
- ¼ cup macadamia nuts, chopped
- 3 tablespoons sugar-free sweetener
- 2 tablespoons raw unsweetened cocoa powder
- Whipped coconut cream

## *Directions:*

1. Place all Ingredients into a blender and blend on high until smooth and creamy.

2. Divide evenly between 4 "mocktail" glasses and top with whipped coconut cream, if desired.

3. Add a cocktail umbrella and toasted coconut for added flair.

4. Enjoy your delicious Choco-nut smoothie!

**_Nutrition_**_:_ 12g Carbohydrates; 3g Protein; 199 Calories

# Pineapple & Strawberry Smoothie

**_Preparation Time:_** 7 minutes

**Cooking Time**: *0 minute*

**Serving**: *2*

## Ingredients:

- 1 cup strawberries
- 1 cup pineapple, chopped
- ¾ cup almond milk
- 1 tablespoon almond butter

## _Directions:_

1. Add all Ingredients to a blender.
2. Blend until smooth.
3. Add more almond milk until it reaches your desired consistency.
4. Chill before serving.

**_Nutrition:_** 255 Calories; 39g Carbohydrate; 5.6g Protein

# Cantaloupe Smoothie

**Preparation Time:** 11 minutes

**Cooking Time**: *0 minute*

**Serving**: *2*

## Ingredients:

- ¾ cup carrot juice
- 4 cups cantaloupe, sliced into cubes
- Pinch of salt
- Frozen melon balls
- Fresh basil

## Directions:

1. Add the carrot juice and cantaloupe cubes to a blender. Sprinkle with salt.
2. Process until smooth.
3. Transfer to a bowl.
4. Chill in the refrigerator for at least 30 minutes.

5. Top with the frozen melon balls and basil before serving.

*Nutrition:* 135 Calories; 31g Carbohydrate; 3.4g Protein

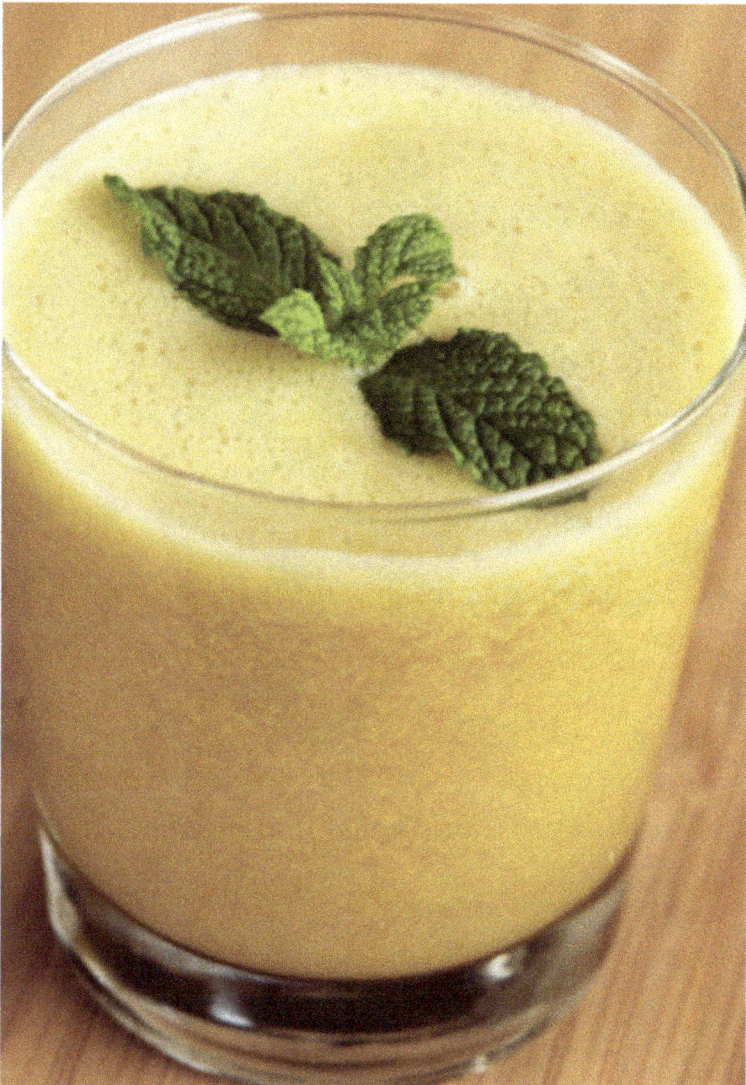

# Berry Smoothie with Mint

***Preparation Time:*** 7 minutes

**Cooking Time***: 0 minute*

**Serving***: 2*

## Ingredients:

- ¼ cup orange juice
- ½ cup blueberries
- ½ cup blackberries
- 1 cup reduced-fat plain kefir
- 1 tablespoon honey
- 2 tablespoons fresh mint leaves

## Directions:

1. Add all the Ingredients to a blender.
2. Blend until smooth.

***Nutrition:*** 137 Calories; 27g Carbohydrate; 6g Protein

# Green Smoothie

**_Preparation Time:_** 12 minutes

**Cooking Time**_: 0 minute_

**Serving**_: 2_

## Ingredients:

- 1 cup vanilla almond milk (unsweetened)
- ¼ ripe avocado, chopped
- 1 cup kale, chopped
- 1 banana
- 2 teaspoons honey
- 1 tablespoon chia seeds
- 1 cup ice cubes

## _Directions:_

1. Combine all the Ingredients in a blender.
2. Process until creamy.

***Nutrition:*** 343 Calories; 14.7g Carbohydrate; 5.9g Protein

# Banana, Cauliflower & Berry Smoothie

***Preparation Time:*** 9 minutes

**Cooking Time**: *0 minute*

**Serving**: *2*

## Ingredients:

- 2 cups almond milk (unsweetened)
- 1 cup banana, sliced
- ½ cup blueberries
- ½ cup blackberries
- 1 cup cauliflower rice
- 2 teaspoons maple syrup

## Directions:

1. Pour almond milk into a blender.
2. Stir in the rest of the Ingredients.
3. Process until smooth.
4. Chill before serving.

***Nutrition:*** 149 Calories; 29g Carbohydrate; 3g Protein

# Berry & Spinach Smoothie

**_Preparation Time:_** 11 minutes

**Cooking Time**: *0 minute*

**Serving**: *2*

## Ingredients:

- 2 cups strawberries
- 1 cup raspberries
- 1 cup blueberries
- 1 cup fresh baby spinach leaves
- 1 cup pomegranate juice
- 3 tablespoons milk powder (unsweetened)

## _Directions:_

1. Mix all the Ingredients in a blender.
2. Blend until smooth.
3. Chill before serving.

**_Nutrition:_** 118 Calories; 25.7g Carbohydrate; 4.6g Protein

# Peanut Butter Smoothie with Blueberries

**Preparation Time:** 12 minutes

**Cooking Time***: 0 minute*

**Serving***: 2*


## Ingredients:

- 2 tablespoons creamy peanut butter

- 1 cup vanilla almond milk (unsweetened)

- 6 oz. soft silken tofu

- ½ cup grape juice

- 1 cup blueberries

- Crushed ice


## Directions:

1. Mix all the Ingredients in a blender.

2. Process until smooth.


**Nutrition:** 247 Calories; 30g Carbohydrate; 10.7g Protein

# Peach & Apricot Smoothie

**_Preparation Time:_** 11 minutes

**Cooking Time**: *0 minute*

**Serving**: *2*

## Ingredients:

- 1 cup almond milk (unsweetened)
- 1 teaspoon honey
- ½ cup apricots, sliced
- ½ cup peaches, sliced
- ½ cup carrot, chopped
- 1 teaspoon vanilla extract
- 

## _Directions:_

1. Mix milk and honey.
2. Pour into a blender.
3. Add the apricots, peaches and carrots.
4. Stir in the vanilla.

5.  Blend until smooth.


***Nutrition:*** 153 Calories; 30g Carbohydrate; 32.6g Protein

# Tropical Smoothie

***Preparation Time:*** 8 minutes

**Cooking Time***: 0 minute*

**Serving***: 2*

## Ingredients:

- 1 banana, sliced
- 1 cup mango, sliced
- 1 cup pineapple, sliced
- 1 cup peaches, sliced
- 6 oz. nonfat coconut yogurt
- Pineapple wedges

## *Directions*:

1. Freeze the fruit slices for 1 hour.
2. Transfer to a blender.
3. Stir in the rest of the Ingredients except pineapple wedges.

4.  Process until smooth.

5.  Garnish with pineapple wedges.

**_Nutrition:_** 102 Calories; 22.6g Carbohydrate; 2.5g Protein

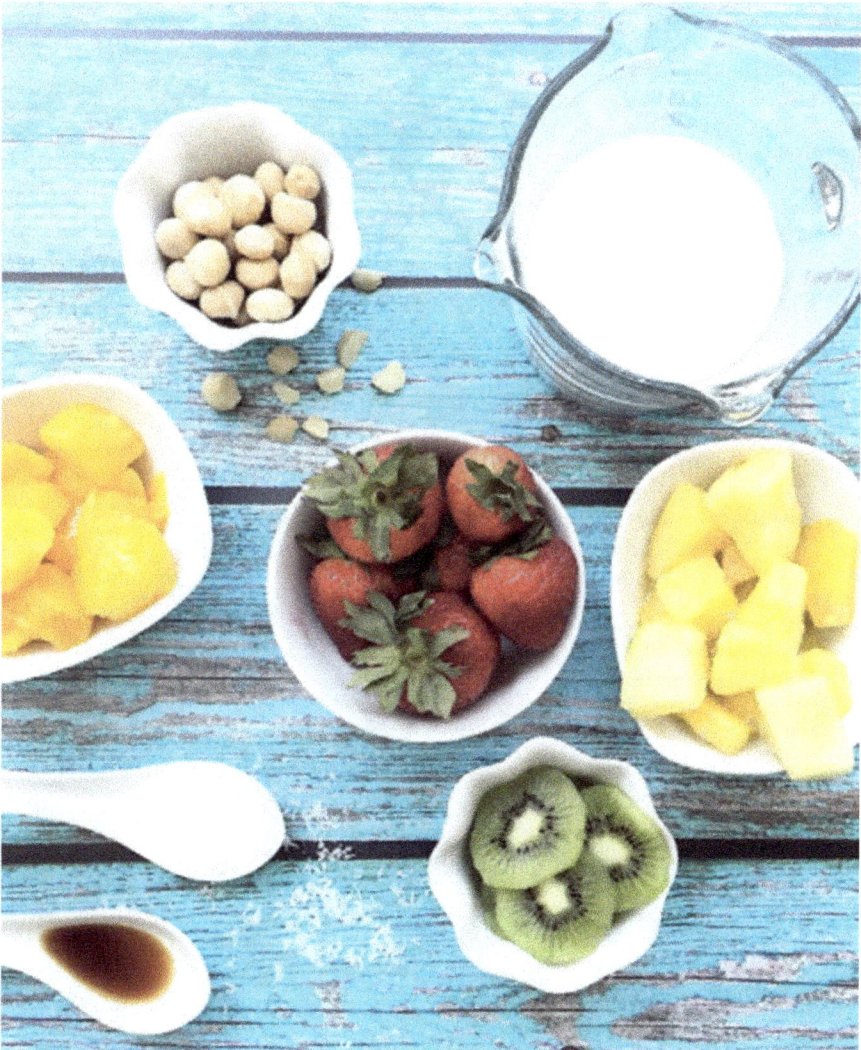

www.ingramcontent.com/pod-product-compliance
Lightning Source LLC
Chambersburg PA
CBHW050745030426
42336CB00012B/1672